EVERYDAY YOGA FOR CHRISTIANS

EVERYDAY YOGA FOR CHRISTIANS

*Seven Simple Steps
to
Victorious Living*

by
ERIC W. HAYDEN, M.A.

JUDSON PRESS, Valley Forge

First Edition 1966
© Eric W. Hayden, 1966
Arthur James Limited of Evesham, Worcs., England
Second Printing, 1972
Judson Press Edition, 1972

International Standard Book No. 0-8170-0555-2
Library of Congress Catalog Card No. 77-181561

BIBLE QUOTATIONS

Scripture sources in this book have been omitted so that the reader may concentrate upon the physical benefits of the various exercises and the extracts quoted. The reader will thus be freed from any additional task.

Except where otherwise stated, the Bible quotations are from the Authorised or King James's version.

Printed in the U.S.A.

CONTENTS

INTRODUCTION

Dr. R. L. Armitstead, M.B., Ch.B.

I AM PRIVILEGED to introduce the Rev. Eric W. Hayden's book *Everyday Yoga for Christians* because I am convinced it is a valuable contribution to the spiritual, mental and physical health of the individual.

The human body is a complex system of intricate muscles working individually or together, usually under the control of the brain. Sometimes it is possible for a muscle to work without the control of the brain, as when an arm is reflexly removed from a painful stimulus, before the pain has registered in the mind; but it is also possible for the brain to control that arm when it is aware that there is going to be a stimulus.

The muscles of the body have to be kept in training if they are to be efficient, and all movements, both single or complicated, can only be done well with exercise and repetition. Exercise promotes strength in the muscles concerned. This can be observed in the professional weight-lifter or the trained athlete. Likewise lack of exercise leads to weakness in the musculature, which, for example, is obvious in the flabbiness of the boxer who has ceased training. It is impossible for the athlete to run a mile in under four minutes without rigorous training, and he accomplishes this with exercise of the correct nature. Similarly, complicated movements of the fingers and hands, as in the case of a violinist or pianist, can only be produced without fatigue if exercise is carried out regularly.

Naturally it is impossible for the middle-aged man to maintain a standard of muscular efficiency equivalent to that of a young man, but it is possible for individuals of *every age* to obtain a physical standard of health by regular exercise. The manual worker of fifty must be physically fitter than the office worker of the same age, but there is nothing to prevent that office worker from reaching a high physical standard by regular exercise in his spare time. I remember well a doctor over fifty years of age who swam two lengths of a swimming pool, *underwater*, every day! He maintained a high standard of fitness by regular exercise.

But regular exercise is not necessarily the only factor in obtaining or maintaining physical fitness. We humans are given a brain which not only co-ordinates our muscles during exercise but controls our desire, or otherwise, to exercise. The doctor could have omitted his underwater swimming for two or three days because the water was too cold or he was overtired, but he would have found his ability to carry out his exercise more difficult on resuming it. He had therefore to discipline his mind to continue his exercise. The athlete might relax his training because he is told that his physical condition was "good enough," and it is only because his brain desires the best from his body that he strives just a little harder. The desire to do one's best creates a mental discipline to control one's exercising capacity.

Most of us are unable to achieve high physical prowess, but we can maintain a reasonable physical standard if we have the mental discipline to do so. It is so much easier to take the easy way out at times, to sit back in front of a warm fire and watch television! The extra effort required to do anything is a product of mental activity, and this exercise is good for the mind, good for the character, and good for the body in general. The more we discipline our minds the faster and more efficient our mental reactions become, so muscle control becomes more acute. We are able to think ahead, so we are mentally in advance of what we propose to do. There is, therefore, a building-up of mental and physical ability all the time, and this leads to a conscious satisfaction and relaxation. There is a peace of mind as a result of one's achievements.

But the human mind is capable of greater things: of deciding between right and wrong, between love and hate, and the ability to exercise faith in God. Having achieved a faith in God, the mind is then governed by an external influence so that the discipline and exercise of the body can be further controlled. Without this influence the mind could decide to use the body for good or evil, but with it there is ensured the use of the body for the benefit of mankind and for the glory of God. The peace of mind and relaxation obtained from our mental-physical efforts now enable us to think quietly about our Creator, what He means to us, and what are His designs for us.

We have been given by God a precious gift. God has entrusted us with a mind and a body to use for His glory, and surely that is our purpose here on earth. We should be conscious of our responsibility and, with faith in His designs, should keep alert and fit so that we are able to use mind and body to their fullest extent in carrying out His purposes for us.

Mr. Hayden has written this book to help us, and I am sure it will prove of great value to the thinking Christian.

R.L.A.

Chapter 1

WHY BE AFRAID?

MANY CHRISTIANS are afraid of Yoga. This fear stems from ignorance or misunderstanding. Because Yoga is known to be a Hindu science of bodily and mental control, or a Hindu system of philosophy, many Christians look upon it as heathenish and therefore to be shunned.

Certainly Yoga is not Christian. The traditional founder of Yoga lived about three centuries before Christ. Nevertheless there are many pre-Christian and post-Christian things in life which the Christian "takes over" and Christianises for his own benefit. For instance, there are many Christians who indulge in what they call "the gentle art of self-defence." This is usually Judo or Ju Jitsu, although it could be Karate. These are Oriental fighting arts that have spread over the centuries to the countries of the West. Judo was originally a monk's defence against thieves. Buddhist monks in Tibet and China devised this system of self-defence for use against bandits who tried to steal their religious robes. In Judo there are terms used such as Judogi (the Judo costume), Kyu and Dan (grades of proficiency). The art is practised in a hall called a Dojo and on a mat which goes by the name of Shiai-jo. The various techniques of Judo have even longer and more peculiar names, yet many Christians are members of Judo clubs and have learned this oriental method of self-defence, invented by non-Christian monks, and no queries are raised as to whether it is a doubtful pursuit for Christians as is so often the case with Yoga.

Many of the terms used in books on Yoga are unacceptable to Christians; terms like "Universal Spirit," "cosmic consciousness," "regeneration" (which has nothing to do with the Christian concept of being "born again" of the Spirit of God—that is, Christian conversion), "salute to the sun," and so on. But Christians should also remember Yoga's positive emphasis upon certain moral virtues: avoidance of injury to others, truthfulness, forgiveness, compassion, sincerity and so on. All these are also truly Christ-like virtues.

Then again, while the Yoga system of physical culture attracts some Christians as a kind of "keep fit" course, they do not like the semi-nude poses, male or female, that illustrate most books on Yoga. That is why in this book simple line drawings are used; added to which, the directness of a line drawing is far more explanatory than some photographs can be.

The names of the Yoga postures or positions are also foreign-looking and sounding to Western minds, and again for Christians seem pagan or heathenish. These "asanas" or natural movements of the limbs and joints of the human body, the adopting of various postures, bear names like "the Cobra," "the Locust," "the Frog," "the Gokarna," and so forth. But why should Christians neglect a system of breathing that is beneficial and a system of physical culture that will enable them to live and function to a greater degree of perfection just because of foreign, strange-sounding names? For that reason I am going to give the exercises in this book simple, English, descriptive names, while at the same time giving some of the usual Yoga terms so that interested readers who wish to check the exercises with any well-known book on Yoga by a non-Christian may do so.

There are, of course, several branches or types of Yoga, each having its own particular emphasis, and I do not think it is out of place to mention some of them. Hatha Yoga is perhaps the best-known in this country, for it deals with the physical body and its health, development and preservation. By contrast, Raja Yoga deals with the mind, its control and development. Then there is Gnani Yoga, which has to do with love of the Absolute, or God. The Yoga of Pantanjali is a systematized religious discipline which concentrates upon *release* (that is, release from self to the attainment of a higher consciousness). All these branches of Yoga have to some extent this common aim—supreme knowledge and liberation. The word Yoga is related to our English word "yoke"—that is, "union." The Yogi seeks after a union between his true self and the Absolute (his conception of God). Every Yogi believes that the practice of Yoga, whichever branch he adheres to, brings him to a certain spiritual goal. Some students of world religions have tried to find a parallel between the Yogi's conception of the Absolute and the Christian's idea of Christ as the Logos or Word.

The true Yogi, then, endeavours to pass from one mental state into successively higher states, and from one spiritual condition into higher spiritual conditions. Finding certain postures useful or beneficial for this dual purpose, he adopts them regularly, gradually attaining greater facility in so doing. The Yogi thus practises or cultivates moral virtues (truthfulness, abstinence, continence, etc.); he also makes a point of regular worship and meditation (promoting tranquillity, renunciation, liberation, illumination, etc.); and finally, through exercises and postures, he achieves vigour and enthusiasm for living.

Our emphasis in this book will be, of course, on a middle-of-the-road path, a combination of Hatha Yoga, with its physical emphasis, and Gnani Yoga, with its love of the Absolute—the Absolute being in the Christian's case the Supreme God, Creator and Redeemer.

Swami Prabhavananda, in *The Spiritual Heritage of India*, quotes Bhoja as saying: "How rare are the souls who at birth are endowed with minds having an aptitude for Yoga. Most men have to mature slowly as they gradually equip themselves with minds fit for practising it." In the same way, we are not born Christians; we have to experience a spiritual rebirth as described by Jesus Christ Himself in John, chapter 3. This spiritual regeneration or conversion experience must be followed by spiritual growth or development. The practice of Yoga will help the Christian to develop "a healthy mind in a healthy body," as the old Latin tag is translated, and also a healthy soul in a healthy body.

The Christian need have no fears in studying and practising Yoga. Dr. Kurt Koch, in his important books on magic, spiritism and the occult (especially *Between Christ and Satan* and *The Strife of Tongues*), has much maligned Yoga when he instances a young man he once counselled who had run into spiritual trouble because he had gone into states of trance. The Yogi need no more go into a trance than lie upon a bed of nails! In any case, what is so anti-Christian about a trance? There are several instances in the Bible of godly men being in a trance during which God made His will and ways known to them.

Prabhavananda also states: "The primary requirement is faith . . . a conviction in the mind; then a response in the heart. When one has faith, one will *act* on that faith." He also comments: "There must, moreover, be spiritual strenuousness. If there is any sin it is laziness." Many Christians are *lazy*—too lazy to take up the practice of

Yoga, something that will benefit them physically, mentally and spiritually. It is hoped that the reader of this book will be stirred to strenuousness, that mind and heart will be given new impetus and direction. As we become more and more absorbed in God we shall be the better equipped to face the trials and tensions, stresses and distresses of everyday life.

What, then, are the real benefits a Christian may expect from following this Yoga system of breathing and exercising? Writing as a minister of the Gospel, I fully concur with Dr. Martyn Lloyd-Jones's opinion of the full-time Christian ministry, that it is "the most exacting vocation that there is." It is a strain on body, mind and spirit. The whole of a man's nervous system is taxed to the uttermost with preparing and delivering sermons and Bible studies, with pastoral visitation in the home and hospital visitation of the sick. The apostle Paul had the "care of all the churches." The care of *one* church is usually enough for a minister to-day!

Many ministers of the Gospel suffer nervous breakdowns; few escape periods of nervous exhaustion; all seem to develop nervous mannerisms in the pulpit. Some are like "a cat on hot bricks" and go from foot to foot in the pulpit; others put their hands behind their back and clench and unclench their fists or fingers. Tension in the neck is not unknown. In fact most ministers finish Sunday well and truly tired, if not exhausted. Many affirm that they "feel fit for nothing" on a Monday. There are so many committees and auxiliary organisations that it is difficult to keep to a day of rest in every week with regularity, and so the toll of one's health goes on. Yet a few moments spent each day on Yoga exercises could change all that.

I write as one who for several years suffered a "slipped disc." The usual treatments were tried: bed at home, bed in hospital, a plaster jacket, and then a leather and webbing belt. Finally an enlightened doctor manipulated, and suggested a course of exercises. Almost immediately I was able to drive my car again instead of standing up in the corridor of the train. Once more I was able to sit in a comfortable armchair instead of on a sit-up-and-beg wooden chair. I began to do my gardening again, play tennis, swim, and, in fact, carry on as before. But one thing I noticed: if I stopped my exercises for any length of time then my back began to stiffen and I could easily "slip" the disc again.

One day I discovered Yoga, and found that some of the Harley Street doctor's recommended exercises were very similar. As I looked at the rather involved Yoga exercises I thought: "Not with my back." But the Yoga system is such that suppleness comes easily and gradually. In fact my own doctor, who also advocated Yoga exercises, said that he had never been able to touch his toes when a boy, but "after a few weeks of Yoga I could!"

Surely the Christian, whether in full-time service or not, should try to have his body in as peak a condition as possible, for then he is able to serve the Lord Jesus Christ as best as he can.

"But what about the Yoga emphasis upon meditation and contemplation?" someone is sure to ask. Yes, there are those whose conception of Yoga is of a man sitting on the ground cross-legged, silently studying his navel. True the Yogi (a Yogi is a practiser of Yoga) does sit or lie silent and contemplative during or in between exercises. But should not the Christian also "Be still, and know that I am God"? We are too prone to rush madly on our way; we do not stop and meditate sufficiently. Where the Yogi may be instructed to think about the Vital Force and to think of some "bright white light" flowing through nose and finger-tips, the Christian who is relaxing through Yoga can pray, or bring to mind Bible promises and passages. One book on Yoga advocates sitting in the characteristic cross-legged (Lotus) posture whenever television is watched or a novel is read. Then let the Christian read his daily Bible portion in that position!

Thus there need be no disharmony between one's Christian faith and the practice of Yoga exercises. Indeed some Christians take up other physical recreation (such as golf, football, boxing, etc.) that brings them into far greater contact with undesirable, non-Christian activities such as drinking and gambling!

Some may ask, "But does not this conflict with Paul's statement: 'For bodily exercise profiteth little: but godliness is profitable unto all things' " (1 Timothy 4 : 8)? The apostle does not say that there is *no profit at all* in physical exercise. If that were the case then there would be no Christian sportsmen at all. No, Paul is not saying that physical exercise is improper—he is only saying that it can be given an improper place in the Christian's life. We must remember that Paul was writing at a time when bodily exercise was regarded by some as an end in itself (perhaps he had the Essenes in mind). Many non-Christians of that era were devotees of asceticism, and worshipped the body instead of the Maker of the body. These people mortified the body by certain dangerous abstinences and penances, turning physical exercise into a religion in itself. So Paul is only warning against going to extremes. The *New Bible Commentary* (Inter-Varsity Fellowship) points out that a Christian minister must keep himself fit by appropriate nourishment and *exercise*, so that one's devotional life and godly living should benefit. That is the end in view for the Christian, according to Paul (who frequently drew his illustrations from the public games!) and that is what we have in view in this

B

book—not bodily exercise as an end in itself, but as a necessary contribution to spiritual wholeness.

There is, of course, the variant reading of the margin, that bodily exercise profiteth *for a little time*. And with some forms of exercise the benefits *are* of short duration. Since Yoga for the Christian is coupled with prayer and meditation it will not have this short-term quality for these devotional exercises are the continuous practice of the Christian. Christian Yoga will in fact promote, prosper and preserve spiritual well-being.

Here, then, is a simple system of breathing, exercise, relaxation and meditation that will improve the Christian's general well-being—physical, mental, nervous, and spiritual. It can be done without any special equipment or dress, although it is best to loosen all tight clothing (collar and tie, waistcoat and belt), remove watch and spectacles, and take off one's shoes. For the rest, the floor of one's bedroom, perhaps with a folded blanket on it, and an open window for fresh air are all that is required. No set time has to be slavishly followed. The exercises are done as one feels the need. No strain is imposed. If an exercise cannot be done strictly according to the diagram, then we get *as near to it* as possible, and a little nearer each week until perfection is attained. Within six weeks we are at near-perfection with the simple exercises; others will require about twelve months. But all the while benefit will be felt.

No one particular time of day is essential. It may be best to fit in some exercises early in the day (before or after breakfast), others midday (after a short rest after lunch), and others in the early or late evening. Most of the exercises can be done at any time of the day when strain is being felt, and they will relieve it, giving fresh energy and strength to cope with life and all its demands. All that is required is determination.

The Yoga system claims to give greater physical health and strength; it claims to help resistance to various illnesses and afflictions; and it claims to help guard against mental and nervous ill-health. Surely these are not anti-Christian? Indeed, many fanatical Yogis have said for a long time that Yoga has ceased to be a religion, it merely "fulfils all the requirements of an ideal method of physical culture." If that is so, then Christians have nothing to fear.

Our aim, then, is Yoga simplified and Yoga Christianised; simple diagrams and names for the exercises, helpful Scriptures to ponder during relaxation.

"Am I too old to begin?" People of seventy and eighty have begun Yoga exercises and have benefited. There is no need for them to "stand on their heads" (in fact there are very few head-stands in Yoga—far fewer than people imagine) or do the more difficult exercises; the simple ones, combined with the breathing and relaxation, should prove sufficient. Women can become as adept and as agile as men. It is one of the cheapest and easiest ways of slimming, without food fads or gadgets.

Small children of five, six or seven years of age love it and are not too young. Naturally they will pick up some of the postures more easily than older members of the family and will provide an incentive for mother and father to "catch up."

"Won't people think me a weirdie?" They may do if you brag or shout about it. But why talk about it unless you are seriously trying to help another person who is anxious to live more positively and vitally? And simply by living as a Christian should live, even without practising Yoga, people will think you a crank or a fanatic! The apostle Paul was right when he wrote: "We are a spectacle unto the world; we are fools for Christ's sake." So expect to be called "Yogi Bear" by unenlightened people!

To sum up then, physically Yoga promotes flexibility and suppleness of muscles; it strengthens and tones up; it removes tenseness; it promotes vitality, endurance and patience; it improves the blood supply and reduces excessive weight. Mentally it contributes to tranquillity and calmness and a banishment of those things that contribute to many of our anxieties and stresses; those undefinable feelings that so sap energy and vitality. Spiritually, if during the exercises important place is given to contemplation, reflection, meditation, self-examination, adoration, praise and prayer, we shall become more mature, more Christ-like, more loving towards our fellow-men, more desirous of serving them as disciples of Christ. Life will thus have more meaning and purpose. It is up to you!

These benefits, physical, mental and spiritual, we shall carry over into all the activities of everyday life, in the home, at business, or wherever we may be and whatever we may be doing. We shall be helped ourselves, and we shall be of help to others. No wonder it has been said that "twenty minutes of Yoga is worth twenty hours of ordinary exercise"!

Without regard to your age, your lack of previous physical exercise, whether you think you are "in" or "out" of condition, begin these exercises at once. Do not despair if some seem difficult, or if you feel you are not achieving the ultimate, extreme position for the required number of seconds—you will in time, with perseverance and patient practice. Notice there is nothing to buy, no special food, no gadgets or expensive sports equipment— you yourself possess all that is necessary. You have only to find the time and the place—the rest is up to you. Approximately twenty minutes a day is all the time that will be taken—perhaps ten in the morning and ten in the evening—but it will be time well spent.

Nothing should interfere with the Christian's Quiet Time with God each day. Well, if these Yoga exercises are combined with the Quiet Time, then regular contact will be maintained with God and regular exercise of the body will be maintained as well, the one influencing the other. Man, after all, has been created body, mind and spirit. Here is a discipline that incorporates and co-ordinates all three. Body, mind and spirit are exercised, controlled and stilled. The body frequently influences the mind. Sometimes there is a predominance of mind over matter. Always for the Christian the spiritual should be uppermost. Yoga for the Christian will keep each part of tripartite man in proper place, perspective and fitness.

Why be afraid, then? That Christians have been afraid of Yoga until fairly recently is proved by the fact that no book from a Christian standpoint has been written upon the subject before except by a Roman Catholic, a Benedictine monk of the Abbey of Saint-André, Prior of the Monastery of Saint-Benoit at Kansenia, Katanga. He, too, was troubled by Christians who viewed Yoga with suspicion, even scepticism, as well as serious misapprehension. Yet Christians should regard Yoga as a means, an aid, an encouragement towards the essential thing in life —"the imitation of (the) Divine Master."

The Master once said: "I am come to bring . . . life, and *far more life than before*" (John 10: 10, J. B. Phillips). The Christian is one who possesses the "more abundant life" of Christ, having received Him into the life by faith. Through the practice of Christian Yoga we can have "more life than before."

Chapter 2

BREATHING

J OHN FRAZER, writing in the *Reader's Digest*, March 1966, entitled his article "Breathe Right—and Stay Well." He advocated the system of seventy-four-year-old William Knowles, who for many years, by correspondence course and personal counselling, has helped many people, doctors included, to obtain better health and renewed vigour through using their lungs in a correct manner. To live man must breath. Restricted breathing means restricted living.

For the Christian correct breathing should be an important matter, for when God first created man He "breathed into his nostrils the breath of life; and man became a living soul" (Genesis 2: 7). The word there for "breath" is the Hebrew *ruach*, used in Scripture for the Holy Spirit. It seems, then, that when man was created his breath had a twofold connection: with his physical and with his spiritual life. Since man was created "in the image" of God, this inbreathing by Almighty God is significant. It was into man's *nostrils* and not into his *mouth* (we shall see later that all Yoga breathing is nostril breathing), so this was no mere "kiss of life" resuscitation, it was the Divine Life Principle giving physical life and immortality to the soul. Our Lord used this same simple picture when speaking to His disciples about the Holy Spirit. Indeed He "breathed on them, and saith unto them, Receive ye the Holy Spirit" (John 20: 22).

In this smoke-ridden twentieth century, with its diesel fumes, its car and motor-cycle exhaust output, its fogs and smogs, the Christian should be careful to breathe properly, remembering that since the Holy Spirit resides in him he is the Temple of God; his physical body is God's House and must be kept pure and clean. In Scripture "breath" is sometimes connected with the will and the emotions. Actors and public speakers have known for a long time that drawing a few deep breaths before singing or speaking in public has helped to "steady their nerves" or overcome stage fright. For singers and speakers, breathing plays a great part in any system of teaching elocution.

Yoga breathing is *controlled* breathing. We sometimes hear people say that breathing is "natural" and "automatic." So it is. When we were born no-one taught us to breathe—we just breathed, as we later saw, heard and ate without any lessons. But the *way* we breathe affects our bodies, nerves and minds. We have only to try the simple experiment of running upstairs to discover the effect breathing has upon us. To know how to breathe properly, then, is the first requirement for success in Yoga. We must be able to breathe in, hold our breath, breathe out again correctly—while we do the exercises and while we relax. Here are several breathing exercises. Some of them can be practised almost anywhere; others would be embarrassing to practise in a public place, so the bedroom or study is the best place.

EXERCISE 1 *Sit-and-Breathe*

IMPORTANT: All breathing in Yoga is through the nostrils with the mouth closed.

Sitting in a comfortable position on an upright chair, keeping the spine straight, breathe in slowly and deeply while counting five. Hold the breath for a slow count of eight, then slowly and silently exhale while counting eight at the same speed.

After practice the counting should be done in seconds. The best way to gauge seconds is to count out "One–lit–tle–boy, two–lit–tle–boys", making the phrase four distinct syllables. This is a method of counting seconds used with great success by photographers.

Exercise 1 should be done five times, then rest, then another group of five, rest again, and a final group of five deep breaths through both nostrils.

EXERCISE 2 *Cross-legged Breathing*

The second simple exercise is similar to the first but is done sitting cross-legged as children do, keeping the back staight. This time the breathing is done through alternate nostrils. The best way to do this is to rest the second finger lightly on the forehead directly above the nose. The thumb can then close the right nostril while breathing is done through the left; the ring or third finger then closes the left nostril while the thumb is released.

Expelling all air from the lungs, the thumb closes the right nostril and air is inhaled through the left nostril for a slow count of eight. The breath is held for a count of eight, with both thumb and ring finger closing *both* nostrils. Then the air is exhaled through the opposite nostril slowly, and for a count of eight. The exercise begins again with the right nostril, the one from which air has just been exhaled.

Again three groups of five are recommended, with a rest in between each group.

This alternate nostril breathing may also be practised sitting upright in a chair as for Exercise 1.

EXERCISE 3 *Kneel-and-Breathe*

Perform the breathing of Exercise 1 while sitting in the relaxed position as shown in the illustration below instead of sitting in a chair or cross-legged.

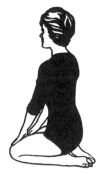

EXERCISE 3: *Kneel-and-Breathe*

Not only is the breathing beneficial but this posture will also help strengthen the legs, thighs and ankles for later Yoga postures that begin in this position.

EXERCISE 4 *Complete Breathing*

Again sit in the cross-legged position. Rest the hands lightly on the knees. Breathe out, emptying the lungs of all air. Draw in breath slowly, filling the abdomen, for a slow count of five. Continue to count five while filling the lower chest. Now press on the knees and lift up the elbows and fill the upper part of the chest with air while counting five slowly. Keeping arms and elbows raised, retain the breath for a count of ten. Then slowly empty the air out in three stages (three counts of five), gradually lowering the arms. Do this five times, rest and repeat.

EXERCISE 5 *Stand-and-Breathe*

Begin by standing upright, feet slightly apart. Bend the knees slightly and lean forward, resting the hands on the thighs. Exhale all air from the lungs; then, without inhaling any air, draw in the adbomen deeply towards the backbone. Keep this position for a slow count of three and then "snap" back the abdomen into its original position. Fill the lungs, exhale again and repeat the abdomen movement. Do this three times in the slight stooping position, then stand upright and rest, breathing easily, before beginning again. Three groups of three should be tried, increasing to five, then ten, and finally fifteen or twenty as time goes on.

All these breathing exercises should be done with closed eyes, the aim being to be as relaxed and calm as possible. The breathing should always be done slowly, smoothly, silently, with any movement of any part of the body carried out slowly and rhythmically. The result will be a loss of flabbiness and a toning-up of the muscles of the stomach and abdomen. Mental and physical fatigue will be greatly alleviated.

Needless to say, these five breathing exercises are not done daily one after the other. They are interspersed with the Yoga postures during a Yoga session, and later a suggested order will be given. Any of them can, and should, however, be practised during the day when the need arises, especially Exercises 1, 2 and 4.

In a relaxed state, with eyes closed, while practising the breathing exercises, the following hymn can be repeated silently. It is possible, with practice, to repeat each line within a period of, say, five seconds, breathing out again for the same period, alternate lines being repeated for the inhalation and the exhalation.

> Breathe on me, Breath of God,
> Fill me with life anew,
> That I may love what Thou dost love,
> And do what Thou wouldst do.
>
> Breathe on me, Breath of God,
> Until my heart is pure,
> Until with Thee I will one will,
> To do or to endure.
>
> Breathe on me, Breath of God,
> Till I am wholly Thine,
> Until this earthly part of me
> Glows with Thy fire divine.
>
> Breathe on me, Breath of God,
> So shall I never die,
> But live with Thee the perfect life
> Of Thine eternity.

This concentration on correct breathing will not only bring about a sense of physical well-being but will impress upon the mind the affinity that there is between the creature and the Creator, man and his Maker. In the words of William Wordsworth, we shall become "a being breathing thoughtful breath."

Chapter 3

RELAXATION

Relaxation is a comparatively modern term. It is not used in the Bible, nor is there any quotation from classical English literature listed in the *Oxford Dictionary of Quotations*. The *idea* of relaxation, however, *is* a Biblical one. It is inherent in the frequently used word "rest." God "rested" on the seventh day (Genesis 2: 2) after His great creative acts. The word means "to cease or desist." According to the writer of the Letter to the Hebrews, the people of God should enjoy a similar "sabbath rest" (Hebrews 4: 9), but not just one day a week—"a sabbath-life" (Wescott's *Epistle to the Hebrews*). There is no suggestion that this rest is reserved for heaven; rather it is to be experienced and enjoyed here and now, although it will reach perfection in heaven.

The Lord Jesus Christ's promise to weary men and women was: "Come unto me, all ye that labour and are heavy laden, and I will give you rest" (Matthew 11: 28). This rest is real "relief, release, and satisfaction to the soul" (Inter-varsity Fellowship's *New Bible Dictionary*). Yet how many Christians know this rest, living as they do in a world of hurry and bustle, each day one mad rush for commuters to our big cities. In our church life we have a multiplicity of meetings and so we hurry to them, "going the rounds" of rallies, committees, conventions, assemblies, and a whole host of "special events." It is possible to be far too busy in the Christian life, *doing* instead of *being*, so losing our Christian attunement with God Who is the Source of all peace and true rest.

Thus contemplation and meditation play a great part in relaxation, for true relaxation is relaxation of the mind and spirit as well as of the body. By placing the body in the right position it helps the mind and spirit to relax with it; it makes it easier for the Christian to think of God with adoring wonder, losing himself and his strains and stresses by contemplating the "peace of God which passeth all understanding" (Philippians 4: 7).

As many Christians are afraid of relaxation, feeling guilty that they are not up-and-doing, so are they chary of contemplation and meditation. These attitudes have been far too long associated with the mystic or the monk. Contemplation and relaxation have been relegated to the monastery or the nunnery. They need to be incorporated into our daily living, so that jagged nerves are "mended" and frayed tempers are "cured," the whole of man (body, mind and spirit) becoming "in tune" with God.

Few people know how to relax in this way. Few find the time to relax. Many think that an ordinary night's sleep is relaxation, or a game of golf, or an evening watching television. But true relaxation is a conscious "letting go," so that tensions are released. Sometimes this tension "catches" people in the head (back or front), the back of the neck, the calves of the legs, the soles of the feet, and can be quite crippling and incapacitating while it lasts. Relaxation can result in a "renewing of the mind" (Romans 12: 2), which then affects these physical symptoms and brings release. There are two "mechanical" aids which help towards achieving this inner state of relaxation, both of which can and should be incorporated within the scheme of Yoga relaxation exercises set out in the following pages.

First, it is helpful to have some of the curtains of the room drawn or the electric light shaded so that the room is in "half-light." An interesting vase or other ornament is then placed in a position where it can be seen without strain. The eyes slowly trace the pattern on the vase until the mind is calm and reflective, the eyes beginning to become heavy as though sleepy. From then on it is helpful to imagine some delightful scene that has happy associations: a favourite holiday spot, a picnic place in the country, and so on. Think of the blue sky, the colour of the water, the green fields, the trees, flowers, sandy shore, and all else that makes up the scene. Imagine you are there with nothing to do except relax—you will then be relaxed! These hints were given to me by a well-known Christian Harley Street doctor. His system of creating a relaxed mind can be used in bed when sleep will not come: it is an excellent cure for insomnia.

True Yoga relaxation can be practised standing, sitting or lying down. Perhaps the method most prevalent in people's minds is the special sitting posture of Yogis. In our section on breathing we have referred to sitting cross-legged. This is a natural position for children, as a visit to any primary school will reveal—they all sit like that in the schoolroom as they listen to their teachers. They also sit like that between exercises when doing physical education. So it is natural for Eastern children to sit in what is called the Yoga "Lotus" position (we shall continue to call it the cross-legged position).

At first you may be able to sit with the legs crossed only like a primary child. Even this position is most relaxing, and should be practised for as long as possible. If you are unused to sitting like this you may, every now and again, stretch out your legs and massage knees, calves or ankles, then re-adopt the position.

Later on you should try this:

EXERCISE 6 *Cross-Legged Relaxation*

Sit in the cross-legged position, then gently lift up one foot and place it in the knee-fold of the other leg. Technically, in Yoga, this is known as the "Half-Lotus". After placing the foot, let your hands rest lightly on your knees. By sitting on a small cushion help is received in the initial stages.

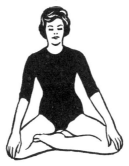

EXERCISE 6: *Cross-Legged Relaxation*

After some weeks (or it may take months—according to your age and suppleness) tuck the other foot up under and place in the oppositive knee-fold—this is now the full cross-legged position, and again the hands rest lightly on the knees.

The eyes are closed when either position is adopted; and whereas the non-Christian Yoga has been advised to let his mind go blank or perhaps meditate on some vital force, the Christian will contemplate God and the wonders of His universe, repeating to himself such verses of Scripture as:

To him who sits upon the throne and to the Lamb be blessing and honour and glory and might for ever and ever. (R.S.V.)

Now unto the blessed and only Sovereign, the King of Kings and Lord of lords, who alone has immortality and dwells in unapproachable light, whom no man has ever seen or can see; to him be honour and eternal dominion. (R.S.V.)

Now to him who by the power at work within us is able to do far more abundantly than all that we ask or think, to him be glory in the Church and in Christ Jesus to all generations, for ever and ever. (R.S.V.)

O God, Thou art my God: early will I seek Thee, my soul thirsteth for Thee. My flesh longeth for Thee . . . to see Thy power and Thy glory.

God is our refuge and strength: a very present help in trouble. Therefore will not we fear though the earth be removed, and though the mountains be carried into the midst of the sea.

Be still and know that I am God: I will be exalted among the nations, I will be exalted in the earth.

Have mercy upon me, O God, according to Thy loving-kindness: according unto the multitude of Thy tender mercies blot out my transgressions. Wash me throughly from mine iniquity, And cleanse me from my sin.

Adoration of God, confession of sin, petition for one's own spiritual needs, intercession on behalf of others—all these can be practised while sitting in the cross-legged position. In between these various "parts" of worship the legs can be crossed in the opposite direction.

EXERCISE 7 *Stand-and-Relax*

In between Yoga postures rest should be taken in a standing position when one standing posture leads on to another in that position. In between sitting or kneeling postures rest will be taken in the cross-legged position. When postures that require lying on one's back are adopted, rest will be taken lying flat. Thus relaxation in a standing position must be practised next.

Learn to stand limp, with arms, hands, wrists, fingers all loose. Let the shoulders go slack. Try to think that the legs and feet are not part of you; then they will not tire because you are standing on them. Breathe gently and easily, not deeply. Close your eyes and repeat to yourself such Scriptural sentences as:

Now to Him who is able to keep you from falling and to present you without blemish before the presence of His glory with rejoicing, to the only God, our Saviour, through Jesus Christ our Lord, be glory, majesty, dominion, and authority, before all time and now and for ever. (R.S.V.)

Or quote to yourself some such hymn or chorus as:

Leaning, leaning (lean on Jesus),
Safe and secure from all alarms;
Leaning, leaning (lean on Jesus),
Leaning on the everlasting arms.

Or:

In thy weakness, in thy peril,
Raise to heaven a trustful call;
Strength and calm for every crisis
Comes by telling Jesus all!

Or:

When I fear my faith will fail,
Christ will hold me fast;
When the tempter would prevail,
He can hold me fast.

c

With the eyes shut, slight swaying movement may be experienced at first, but this will be overcome as you practise relaxation in this standing position between postures. Needless to say, relaxation in the standing position is not held for as long as relaxation sitting or lying down—it is merely a question of quiet rest between standing postures.

EXERCISE 8 *Lie-and-Relax*

Relaxation lying down is the ultimate in relaxation. While what we describe here is for use in a daily Yoga session, it can also be practised in bed at night and will induce sleep quicker than "counting sheep" or drinking patent health foods.

Lie on the floor on your back. Let your arms flop to your sides, about one foot from your body. Your heels should also be about a foot apart, toes pointing outwards. Place the palms of the hands uppermost, open, and fingers relaxed. Close your eyes and let scalp, forehead, eyelids, mouth, jaw, shoulders, arms, back, legs, feet, toes, go as limp as possible. Sometimes you should tighten the scalp, hands, and so on, and deliberately "let them go" to achieve this looseness and utter relaxation. Always begin at the head and work down to the feet.

Complete relaxation having been attained, feeling sleepy and yet not asleep, let a sense of well-being come over you as you repeat Bible promises and hymns applicable to this state. For example, begin with two prayer hymns:

> May the Word of God dwell richly
> In my heart from hour to hour,
> So that all may see I triumph
> Only through His power.

And:

> O Master, let me walk with Thee
> In lowly paths of service free;
> Tell me Thy secret; help me bear
> The *strain of toil*, the *fret of care*.

Or perhaps:

> Speak, Lord, in the stillness,
> While I wait on Thee;
> Hushed my heart to listen
> In expectancy.

Make this period of relaxation a time of real peace—peace with God, peace with oneself, and peace with one's fellow men. If you are relaxing in the morning (many people find this the best time for a Yoga session), then here is a helpful hymn:

> I met God in the morning.
> When my day was at its best,
> And His Presence came like sunrise,
> Like a glory in my breast.
>
> All day long the Presence lingered;
> All day long He stayed with me,
> And we sailed in perfect calmness
> O'er a very troubled sea.
>
> So I think I know the secret
> Learned from many a troubled way;
> You must seek Him in the morning
> If you want Him through the day.

This lying-flat relaxation can become an exercise in itself—say a period of ten minutes at a time. Or it can be just one minute of rest in between certain Yoga postures which we shall learn. If it becomes a ten-minute period at some time during the day, then the following Scriptures are helpful to recall while relaxing (remember that Jesus Christ promised His Holy Spirit "would bring to remembrance", so rely on the Spirit to do just that, recalling for you precious promises from His word):

The heavens declare the glory of God; and the firmament sheweth His handywork.

Glory to God in the highest, and on earth peace, good will toward men.

We love Him, because He first loved us.

For He knoweth our frame; He remembereth that we are dust.

Behold the fowls of the air: for they sow not, neither do they reap, nor gather into barns; yet your heavenly Father feedeth them. Are ye not much better than they?

That Christ may dwell in your hearts by faith; that ye, being rooted and grounded in love, may be able to comprehend with all saints what is the breadth, and length, and depth, and height; and to know the love of Christ, which passeth knowledge, that ye might be filled with all the fullness of God.

Eye hath not seen, nor ear heard, neither have entered into the heart of man, the things which God hath prepared for them that love Him.

As with the breathing exercises (which are meant to be practised one after the other but interspersed between Yoga postures), so these relaxation positions are to be incorporated within the Yoga scheme of exercises.

The true Yogi believes in three stages in the process of relaxation: Concentration, Meditation, and Absorption. By following the suggestions given at the beginning of this chapter, and then by practising the exercises that follow, these three stages will be reached.

The final state, Absorption, the culmination of relaxation, is a spiritual illumination of the mind whereby the relaxed person is able, "outside of himself," to enter into deep communion with God. This, surely, is what the apostle Paul meant when he said: "I knew a man in Christ above fourteen years ago, (whether in the body, I cannot tell; or whether out of the body, I cannot tell: God knoweth;) such an one caught up to the third heaven . . . he was caught up into paradise, and heard unspeakable words, which it is not lawful for a man to utter" (2 Corinthians 12: 2, 4). There, in the "third heaven," relaxed, contemplative, meditative, communing with God, we are far and away above the world of noise and tumult, with all the attendant strain and stress, worry and anxiety. Such a state of relaxation, in the words of Hamlet, " 'Tis a consummation devoutly to be wish'd." The wish may be fulfilled through the practice of Yoga relaxation exercises, combined with reliance upon the ministry of the Holy Spirit, for the kind of meditation and contemplation that is required for utter and complete relaxation cannot come entirely from oneself. Discipline and exercise are but a positive way. The power of the Holy Spirit must, with quiet magnetic force, draw our mind and spirit in the desired direction, Godwards.

Chapter 4

POSTURES

D R. MARTYN LLOYD-JONES of Westminster Chapel, London, has done great service to Christians by preaching a comprehensive series of sermons on Ephesians, chapter 6. In one sermon he points out how the apostle Paul emphasises several times that the Christian must "stand." The exhortation is given four times. Dr. Lloyd-Jones comments: "It is a very wonderful word, it is a kind of 'order for the day.' This is the great appeal that comes to Christian people."

Many Christians feel weak, physically and spiritually. Some are full of self-pity of a crippling kind. Others feel sorry for themselves all the time, discouraged and complaining. God does not seem to be fulfilling His promises, giving us a sense of strength, vitality and victory. Sometimes we feel alarmed, frightened by life and all its difficulties and hardships. We become half-hearted and uncertain.

The apostle's remedy is to "stand"! He advocates a stance, not a slouch. Dr. Lloyd-Jones puts it: "Do not lean against your post; stand at your post." When so many people in the world are bowed down by worries and anxieties; when they go under because their weight of difficulties grows too great; then it is that the Christian should be able to stand upright as a true testimony to the upholding-power of God.

Christianity is manly, not namby-pamby. We are to

"Quit you like men. Be strong." We must be "more than conquerors." Our stance or posture before the world must be upright. This is the Christianity of the hymn-writers. How many of their hymns urge us to "Stand up, stand up for Jesus," or "Stand then in His great might"? We are expected to stand up for the truth and that which is right; to stand out against the moral and social evils of our time; to stand against oppression and racial discrimination. But all our moral and spiritual stances will be as nothing unless we can be looked upon as standing in a physical sense as well. The world will always consider the inner from the outer; it will always judge the inner man, with his convictions, from his outward appearance.

We come then to further Yoga postures, the various stances and exercises that, practised daily, will promote suppleness and vitality. They are given here in order of easiness of learning, and in such an order that they lead from one to another for promoting a progressive feeling of betterment throughout the entire body. As the body begins to feel more supple and youthful, so the mind and and nervous system, and the spiritual life, will also benefit.

EXERCISE 9 *The Leg-Pull*

We begin with exercises done in a sitting position, and in our final daily plan of exercises it will be seen how breathing and relaxation fit into this scheme in the same position.

For Exercise 9, as shown on the next page, we sit on the floor with legs extended in front of us. Slowly raising our arms until level with our shoulders, we then reach forward and grasp our legs firmly as near to the ankle as possible. (See Fig. 1.) We then pull at our legs, bending our backs, and dropping our head down towards our knees. When we have gone as far as we can (we shall be able to go farther each week with increasing suppleness) we remain in that position for ten seconds, keeping our eyes closed. (See Fig. 2.)

It is helpful to bend the elbows slightly outwards to help the head come nearer to the knees. After a few weeks this position can be maintained for fifteen instead of ten seconds.

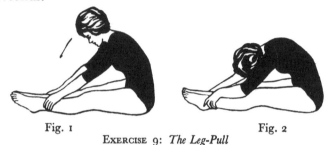

Fig. 1   Fig. 2

EXERCISE 9: *The Leg-Pull*

After holding the position for the prescribed time we sit up straight, rest for a few moments, then repeat. This exercise is done three times.

It is helpful to have a kitchen timer, or one of those recent motorist's pocket parking timers, close by while doing some of these exercises. The timer can be set for the prescribed number of seconds, which eliminates counting so prayers can be said, or passages of Scripture repeated, during the restful part of the exercise. During the Leg-Pull exercise it is helpful to repeat words such as:

Is not the life more than meat, and the body than raiment?

Seek ye first the kingdom of God, and His righteousness; and all these things shall be added unto you.

Or:

O holy God, I ask this boon of Thee:
Be mine, in truth, a soul that worships; free

From all profane and trivial thoughts, and filled
With reverential faith; a soul all stilled
In hush of awe; since Thou, the God most high,
To lowly, contrite men, art ever nigh.

Exercise 10 *The Leg-Flop*

Again sitting upright with legs in front of the body, stretched out fully, slowly draw them towards you, letting your knees come wide apart but holding your soles together with your hands, as in Figure 1. Pulling upwards on the feet, let your knees and thighs flop towards the floor as far as they will go (they will go farther each week until they rest on the floor.) (See Fig. 2 below.)

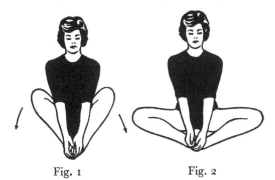

Fig. 1   Fig. 2

Exercise 10: *The Leg-Flop*

Keep this position, with eyes closed, for a count of fifteen seconds. If you set your timer before doing this exercise (which is done three times with a rest in between each one), then you can concentrate upon peaceful, helpful words such as these:

Now, life itself is worship; for in me
The Christ is dwelling, and I live to Thee;
Thine all-pervading presence is made known
Within the soul; I cannot be alone,

> For Thou, to me, art life; and I adore
> Thy matchless grace, and worship evermore.

Or:

> Whatsoever things are true, whatsoever things are honest,
> whatsoever things are just, whatsoever things are pure,
> whatsoever things are lovely, whatsoever things are of
> good report, if there be any virtue, and if there be any
> praise, think on these things.

EXERCISE 11 *The Backward Bend*

Now sit on your heels, your knees together in front of you. Do not curl up your toes beneath you; let them point out behind you, as in Figure 1 below. Place your hands on the floor beside you and one at a time "walk" them behind you, palms flat on the floor, leaning back as you do so. When you are leaning back as far as you can go, let your head lean back, at the same time pushing your abdomen and chest out and upwards. Looking upwards at the ceiling, keeping the eyes open this time, count ten seconds, increasing to fifteen, then twenty as the weeks go by (See Fig. 2 below.)

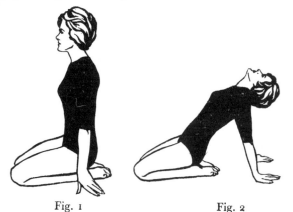

Fig. 1   Fig. 2

EXERCISE 11: *The Backward Bend*

At the end of the count "walk" your hands forward and sit once again on your heels for a rest. Repeat this exercise three times.

As you look up at the ceiling, see beyond it or through it, heavenwards, repeating to yourself such texts or verses as the following:

> God be in my head,
> And in my understanding;
> God be in mine eyes,
> And in my looking;
> God be in my mouth,
> And in my speaking;
> God be in my heart,
> And in my thinking;
> God be at mine end,
> And at my departing.

Or:

Where your treasure is, there will your heart be also.

Be of good cheer; I have overcome the world.

When I consider thy heavens, the work of thy fingers, the moon and the stars, which thou hast ordained; what is man, that thou art mindful of him? and the son of man, that thou visitest him?

From sitting postures we now turn to those standing upright.

EXERCISE 12 *On Your Toes*

Standing with feet about one foot apart, raise your arms in front of you until they are shoulder high. Extend your fingers and keep your thumbs together. (See Fig. 1 on next page.) Raising yourself as high as you can on your toes, turn yourself to the left until you are at right angles from the waist. You will wobble a bit at first, but persevere until you can keep your balance. Keep your eyes open all the while. Remain in the extreme position for ten, then later fifteen and finally twenty seconds as you become more and more proficient. (See Fig. 2 below.)

Now return to the forward position and slowly lower your arms and feet until you are standing upright and still with arms at your sides. Rest and repeat the exercise,

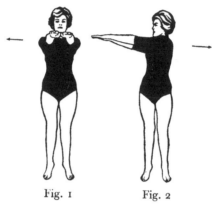

Fig. 1   Fig. 2

EXERCISE 12: *On Your Toes*

but to the right. The exercise is not completed until two turns have been made to the left and two to the right (Fig. 2). At first it will be wise not to think, pray or repeat verses—concentrate on not overbalancing, not wobbling, but remaining still on the toes at all times. When proficiency has been reached (in a matter of six or eight weeks) repeat the following, making sure you keep your eyes at all times on your thumbs:

The steps of a good man are ordered by the Lord; and He delighteth in his way. Though he fall, he shall not be utterly cast down: for the Lord upholdeth him with His hand.

Put on the whole armour of God, that ye may be able to stand against the wiles of the devil.

When ye stand praying, forgive, if ye have aught against any: that your Father also which is in heaven may forgive you your trespasses.

Trust ye in the Lord for ever: for in the Lord Jehovah is everlasting strength.

Or:

Stretch forth, O Lord, Thy mercy over Thy servant, even the right hand of heavenly help, that I may seek Thee with my whole heart, and obtain what I rightly ask for, through Jesus Christ our Lord (Ancient Collect).

Or:

O Lord, who knowest me to be set in the midst of so many dangers, that by reason of the frailty of my nature I cannot always stand upright: grant to me such strength and protection as may support me in all dangers, and carry me through all temptation, through Jesus Christ our Lord (Liturgy).

EXERCISE 13 *Arm-and-Leg Triangle*

Again stand with legs about one foot apart, hands at side. Raise the right arm upwards into a "Hitler" salute. Put all your weight on your right foot. Now bend back your left leg from the knee and grasp your toes with the left hand. (See Fig. 1 on the next page.) Bring the "saluting" arm back farther, lean your head back slightly, and look up at the ceiling with your eyes open. (See Fig. 2 on the next page.)

Come back to the standing position, rest and repeat with the opposite limbs. Do the exercise twice on each leg, for a count of ten seconds. Once more you will wobble until you have practised for some weeks, so concentrate on remaining steady and counting the seconds. Do not

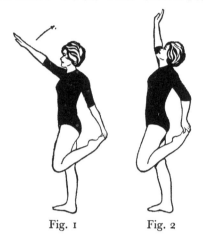

Fig. 1   Fig. 2

EXERCISE 13: *Arm-and-Leg Triangle*

pray, meditate or repeat any helpful verses until you are proficient. You may have to practise near a wall at first in case you lose your balance. When you can do this posture without fear of falling, then use some, or all, of the following:

> The servant of the Lord must not strive; but be gentle unto all men.
>
> Thanks be unto God, which always causeth us to triumph in Christ.
>
> As thy days, so shall thy strength be.
>
> Thy word is a lamp unto my feet, and a light unto my path.
>
> Some trust in chariots, and some in horses: but we will remember the name of the Lord our God.

Or:
> I know not what may soon betide,
> Nor how my wants will be supplied;
> But Jesus knows and will provide.

Though faint my prayers, and cold my love,
My stedfast hope shall not remove
While Jesus intercedes above.

EXERCISE 14 *Chest Expander*

Begin once again by standing upright with arms at the side. This time the feet should be together and *not* apart. Bring the arms up to the front, bending the elbows, chest high. Straighten out the arms and swing them behind you, clasping your hands behind your back. Keep the hands clasped and push backwards with your arms, at the same time looking up at the ceiling with eyes open. Remain like this for five seconds. (See Fig. 1 below.) Then slowly lower your head and shoulders, bending from the waist, still keeping your hands clasped and arms straight. Get the head as close to the knees as possible, pushing forwards with your arms. Remain in this position for ten seconds. (See Fig. 2 below.)

Slowly straighten up, rest and repeat. This exercise is

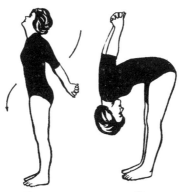

Fig. 1   Fig. 2
EXERCISE 14: *Chest Expander*

done only twice, *not* three times, for it is strenuous and brings the blood to the head in a revitalising way.

For the five seconds looking up (See Fig. 1, previous page) repeat short verses of Scripture such as:

For Thy name's sake lead me and guide me.

Draw nigh to God, and He will draw nigh to you.

Be kindly affectioned one to another with brotherly love.

For the ten seconds head down (See Fig. 2, previous page) meditate on these words:

Labour not to be rich: cease from thine own wisdom.

They that trust in the Lord shall be as Mount Zion, which cannot be removed, but abideth for ever.

Heaven and earth shall pass away: but my words shall not pass away.

Jesus Christ, the same yesterday, and to-day, and for ever.

We have now completed all the exercises from a standing position, so finally we shall practise some from a lying position—some from a prone position on the front, others lying on our back.

EXERCISE 15 *The Upward-Press*

Known by Yogis as "The Cobra," the Upward-Press is begun by lying flat on the floor, face downwards, the head turned to one side, resting the cheek on the floor (which ever side feels the more comfortable). Turning the head face downwards, the forehead resting on the carpet or rug, the exercise begins.

Raise the head and shoulders as far as possible without help from the arms lying at your side. (See Fig. 1 below.) When that position is reached, slide the hands and arms beneath the chest, the fingers of each hand pointing slightly inwards, and push up until the arms are straight. Bend the head back looking towards the ceiling. (See Fig. 2 below.) The extreme position is reached very slowly, and the body remains resting on the floor in the region of the groin.

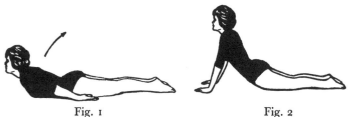

Fig. 1 Fig. 2

EXERCISE 15: *The Upward-Press*

This position is held for ten seconds (working up later to fifteen) and then the arms allow the trunk to be lowered until it is once again self-supporting. The head is lowered to the floor and then turned on one side, the cheek resting on the rug. Rest and relax.

This exercise is *never* repeated straight away; it is always done in conjunction with Exercises 16, 17 and 18, in rotation.

As these are strenuous exercises it is advisable to concentrate on every part of them, especially the time spent in the extreme position, and no prayer or meditation or repetition of Scripture verses is recommended.

EXERCISE 16 *The Leg-Lift*

Again lying on the floor face down, head on one side, we begin the Leg-Lift (known by Yogis as "The Locust")

D

Fig. 1

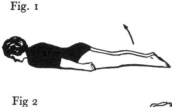

Fig 2

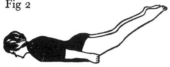

EXERCISE 16: *The Leg-Lift*

by turning the head and resting the chin (not the forehead this time) on the floor. (See Fig. 1.) Clenching the hands by our sides, we press down on the clenched fists and slowly raise both legs as high as they will go. (See Fig. 2.)

If it is easier to lift one leg, lower it, lift the other, lower it, then lift both together, this method may be used. When both legs are raised in the air they must be held in this position for three seconds, then five a few weeks later, until seven is reached. They are lowered slowly and not allowed to drop. Rest with the head on one side and relax. This exercise is not repeated until Exercises 17, 18 and again 15 have been done.

EXERCISE 17 *The Boat*

The Boat posture is known by Yogis as "The Bow." Again the face-down, face-on-one-side, prone position is adopted to begin the exercise. Again the head is turned until the chin is on the floor. Then the legs are bent back at the knees until the arms at the sides can catch hold of them (you may have to take hold of one leg at a time at first) by the instep. (See Fig. 1.)

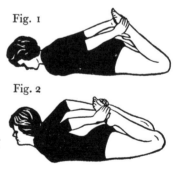

Fig. 1

Fig. 2

EXERCISE 17: *The Boat*

Gradually pull on the legs and at the same time raise head and shoulders until both extremities are clear of the ground and you resemble a small boat. (See Fig. 2 on opposite page.) Hold this position for ten seconds, then lower the legs and then the head. Rest and relax and do not repeat.

EXERCISE 18 *The Neck-Twist*

Lying face downwards, face turned on one side, begin by turning head and raising it to rest against your arms with the fingers intertwined on top of your head. (See Fig. 1 below.) Remain in this restful position for twenty seconds, then place the left hand beneath the chin and, with the help of the right hand on the head, twist the head and neck to the left. (See Fig. 2 below.) Hold this

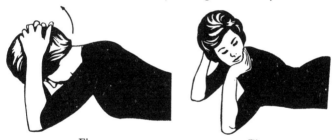

Fig. 1   Fig. 2
EXERCISE 18: *The Neck-Twist*

position for twenty seconds. Return to the first position for twenty seconds, then do the same to the right, with the right hand cupped under the chin. Retain this position for twenty seconds and return to the in-between position for twenty seconds. This is a very restful and relaxing exercise and always follows the previous three, the Up-ward-Press, the Leg-Lift and the Boat (Exercises 15, 16 and 17). Thus these four exercises are done in rotation three times. If it is found more restful, the Neck-Twist can be done in between the Upward-Press and the Leg-Lift, and in between the Boat and the Leg-Lift.

We have completed all lying-down exercises from a face-down position; now we have two to learn from the face-up position—the Plough and the Shoulder-Stand.

EXERCISE 19 *The Plough*

Lying flat on the back with arms at the side, palms downwards, we begin the Plough by pressing down with the hands, at the same time raising the legs into the air, keeping them perfectly straight all the time. (See Fig. 1 below.) Slowly we let them come over our head until they reach the floor behind. (See Fig. 2 below.)

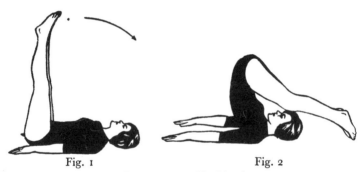

Fig. 1   Fig. 2

EXERCISE 19: *The Plough*

This will not be achieved without considerable practice, so we must for some weeks be content with the legs being parallel with our body. The prone position is returned to by bending the legs at the knees, pressing on the floor with the palms, and swinging the legs back to the floor. Rest and relaxation follow. The extreme position is at first held only for ten to twenty seconds to begin with, working up to one whole minute as the weeks go by. The exercise is done only once and is not repeated. If it appears hard on the head or neck, then a folded towel should be placed beneath the head and the exercise should not be done again until all stiffness is gone.

EXERCISE 20 *The Shoulder-Stand*

Lying on the back once again, with palms down, the hands are pressed hard against the floor and the legs raised straight in the air as in the Plough. But once the legs are in the air the hands and arms are then moved to rest on the hips. (See Fig. 1 below.)

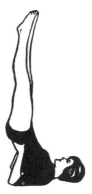

Fig. 1
EXERCISE 20: *The Shoulder-Stand*

The hands push up on the hips until they can support the top of the buttocks. The chin is thus pressed against the chest. The eyes are closed and breathing is slow and deep from the abdomen. The extreme position is held as for the Plough, starting with ten seconds, then twenty, until the position can be held for one minute. Later on the Plough and the Shoulder-Stand will be held for anything up to five minutes.

To regain the prone position the legs are again bent, the arms and hands placed by the side, palms down, and the legs then lowered slowly to the floor. Rest and relaxation are then essential.

As these last two exercises gradually increase in time, it is useless suggesting short passages to recite or meditate upon. Long passages would not be easily remembered, so it is best to use the time for private prayer and meditation. Alternatively, a tape-recorded session of helpful prose and verse might be played, or recorded sacred music with a message of its own. Superimposed on the tape could be timing in seconds or in minutes, and thus the mind need not be preoccupied with counting time. All Yoga exercises are more beneficial when the mind and spirit are in contemplative mood and not too taken up with the technicalities of the exercises.

EXERCISE 21 *Face-down Relaxation*

In between Exercises 15, 16 and 17, performed in rotation, it has been recommended that the Christian Yogi should rest and relax. This face-down relaxation is, in fact, a reversal of the procedure of Exercise 8 (Lie-and-Relax).

Lying prone on the stomach with the face turned to one side, cheek against the rug on the floor, the legs are slightly apart, about one foot to eighteen inches, with the heels leaning outwards. The palms of the hands are upwards. With closed eyes the whole body is made to go limp, from head to feet, as in Exercise 8. Once this is achieved it is advisable to repeat verses of Scripture and pray, remembering that in the Old Testament the great saints of God were frequently "on their faces before the Lord." This is not only the position of relaxation but also of humiliation. In this position we remember that we are nothing and that God is everything. Thus we pray to Him:

> I set my face unto the Lord God, to seek by prayer and supplications, with fasting, and sackcloth, and ashes; and I prayed unto the Lord my God, and made my confession.

> To the Lord our God belong mercies and forgivenesses, though we have rebelled against him.

> O Lord, hear; O Lord, forgive; O Lord, hearken and do; defer not, for thine own sake, O my God.

> If my people, which are called by my name, shall humble themselves, and pray, and seek my face, and turn from their wicked ways; then will I hear from heaven, and will forgive their sin, and will heal their land.

Or:

> Jesus! I am resting, resting
> In the joy of what Thou art;
> I am finding out the greatness
> Of Thy loving heart.
> Thou hast bidst me gaze upon Thee,
> And Thy beauty fills my soul,
> For, by Thy transforming power,
> Thou hast made me whole.

In days when so many people crowd the surgeries of doctors, complaining of nothing more than that they feel "out of condition" or "under par," lacking energy and "drive," who would begrudge twenty or thirty minutes a day practising these exercises designed to rid the body of stiffness, tension, flabbiness and fatness, and give to the Christian the utmost fitness for serving Christ and His Church?

After only a few weeks of practising these postures you will not only *feel* better but others will tell you that you *look* better. If your daily work involves a great deal of sitting, then these exercises are essential to combat the drawbacks of a sedentary occupation. If your job involves much standing, then these postures will strengthen you for such work. In fact the manual worker, the shop assistant, the student, the teacher, the minister of religion, the cabinet minister—those in every walk of life—will be helped by these simple, basic Yoga postures.

Chapter 5

SCHEDULES

"LET ALL THINGS be done decently and in order," wrote the apostle Paul to the Corinthians. Many people's lives are chaotic rather than well-regulated. For Christians this should not be. The Bible reveals Almighty God as a God of order and design. He works to a time-table. This is seen in the creation of the world as recorded in the Book of Genesis, and in the study of prophecy throughout the Bible. As A. C. Ainger, the hymn writer, expressed it:

> God is working His purpose out
> As year succeeds to year.

The Christian is a steward. God has entrusted to him money, possessions, gifts and talents, *and time*. All are to be used in a worthy manner in God's service. Of the Christian's time the Bible says: "Redeeming the time" (Ephesians 5: 16)—that is, we must exercise Christian prudence, using our time wisely and well. "Grasp it" or "buy it up" are better translations of "redeem."

Twenty-one basic Yoga exercises have now been learned. They must now be practised according to a strict schedule, although they will not be practised in the order they have been learned. So far they have been grouped into three sections—sitting, standing and lying positions, for this has been the easiest and most progressive way of learning and remembering them. Now they must be practised regularly each day according to a strict schedule.

"Evening, and morning, and at noon, will I pray," declared the Psalmist. The prophet Daniel opened his window towards Jerusalem "three times a day, and prayed." The Christian life is a disciplined, well-regulated life according to the apostles Peter and Paul. We must set aside time for serious reading and study of the Bible, time for prayer and meditation, time for the service of God to the community, and time for the practice of Yoga. Since, as we have seen, the Christian's Quiet Time (Bible reading, meditation and prayer) can be combined with certain exercises, the amount of time to be devoted to Yoga each day is not excessive.

Two time-tables are given—to be used on alternate days. If time permits, the whole of the exercises can be done in one period of time; but it is better to have two Yoga sessions a day, morning and afternoon or morning and evening, and the letters A.M. and P.M. show a convenient point of division for the two suggested sessions per day.

SCHEDULE I (Monday, Wednesday and Friday)
A.M.
Sit-and-Breathe (Exercise 1)
Stand-and-Breathe (Exercise 5)
The Leg-Pull (Exercise 9)
The Leg-Flop (Exercise 10)
Cross-legged Relaxation (Exercise 6)
On Your Toes (Exercise 12)
Stand-and-Relax (Exercise 7)

P.M.
Chest Expander (Exercise 14)
The Upward-Press ⎫ Exercises 15, 16, and 17 to be
The Leg-Lift   ⎮ done in rotation, with Exercise
The Boat   ⎰ 21 (Face-down Relaxation) at
The Neck-Twist ⎭ end; or Exercise 18 in between 15

and 16, 16 and 17, again ending with No. 21.
Complete Breathing (Exercise 4)

SCHEDULE 2 (Tuesday, Thursday, Saturday)
A.M.
Sit-and-Breathe (Exercise 1)
Cross-legged Relaxation (Exercise 6)
Kneel-and-Breathe (Exercise 3)
The Backward Bend (Exercise 11)
Arm-and-Leg Triangle (Exercise 13)
Stand-and-Relax (Exercise 7)

P.M.
Complete Breathing (Exercise 4)
The Plough (Exercise 19)
Lie-and-Relax (Exercise 8)
The Shoulder-Stand (Exercise 20)
Lie-and-Relax (Exercise 8)
Cross-legged Breathing (Exercise 2)

It will be noticed that all sessions on alternate days begin with a breathing exercise or two. Then a fairly simple exercise follows to promote suppleness before attempting the more difficult exercises. All sessions end with breathing and/or relaxation.

What about Sunday? Sunday, by Divine command, is a day of rest. The main body of exercises is not performed on the Lord's Day. However, for preachers, Sunday-school teachers, choir members, and any others who have Christian service to perform, there is no harm, indeed much benefit will be derived from the breathing and relaxation exercises, especially Nos. 1, 6 and 14.

What happens if a day has to be missed completely during the week? Wherever you are, try to do some of the breathing exercises. But do not worry about missing a day's schedule. The following day fit in as many of the easier exercises of the missed day in order to "limber up", but there is no need to do "a double dose." Yoga is a science or art that helps to combat worry and anxiety, not produce them! So do not worry over a missed day's schedule through business taking you from home, or some other reason. Of course, it is possible to rise a little earlier that morning and fit in some of the exercises! Perhaps business will go all the better for having done so.

It has been said that for the Christian time is not an "abstract problem" but "a created sphere." In other words, time is a God-given commodity appropriate for "given undertakings." The terms "day", "hour", "to-day", "now" occur throughout the Bible with dramatic significance. Yet how many Christians talk of "killing time" or "passing the time"? Time should be taken seriously by the Christian, for one day we shall have to render an account of what we have done with our time; how we have spent it, or wasted it. This is where the Christian Yogi has an advantage over the non-Christian practitioner of Yoga. The Buddhist conception of time is that it is evil. The Christian knows it as a Divine creation, and so he is careful to use his time to the full, faithfully working to a time-table in the secular and the spiritual spheres. The dilatory, undisciplined person will *never* obtain the fullest benefit from Yoga, for he or she will too frequently forget or give up the practice schedules.

As we have seen, it is the duty of every Christian to seek and maintain a healthy body and the schedules of simple basic Yoga as suggested in this chapter will do just that. It is up to you.

Chapter 6

BENEFITS

A COMMON "grace before meat" with Christians is the Psalmist's exhortation in Psalm 103: "Bless the Lord, O my soul, and forget not all His benefits." What numerous benefits we receive from our bountiful heavenly Father! Blessings in the material and temporal, spiritual and eternal spheres, *daily*! While we are often urged to "count our blessing, name them one by one," even if we count quickly two by two or four by four, we cannot make up the sum total.

At the creation of the world God pronounced all things "good." Sometimes God's good gifts are unwisely used, or even abused, and so we live in a world of drunkenness and drug addiction. But God has made many things for the physical benefit of mankind. Some of these "benefits," or Divine blessings, have never been experienced or enjoyed by Christians because they have neglected to accept that which God offers. Being set in their ways, they have not dared to venture out to "pastures new." If only they would take such a step into "fresh fields" they would never want to go back because of the wonderful new experiences and wealth of good things.

Venture and Adventure are two words that many Christians need to include in their vocabulary. Like the disciples, they need to "launch out into the deep." New ways of contact and communion with God must be engaged in; new methods of physical, mental and spiritual fitness must be tried. Christian Yoga is one of these, and those who have taken it up in recent years have often given the following unsolicited testimony: "Tried and found successful." New vitality and energy have been discovered; a more quiet and peaceful way of life has occurred; more regular periods of prayer and meditation have taken place; more freedom from stress and tension has been found. Curiosity and caution having been overcome, the benefits of Yoga have become a source of strength and delight. That which was previously thought of as a philosophy, and a mystic philosophy at that, has been seen to be physical and spiritual—these two benefiting the mental state also.

Great claims have been made by Yogis throughout the years as to the benefits derived from a practice of Yoga. The only real access to these benefits is to "try it and see." The frame of mind with which a person undergoes such a course as the one suggested here will influence the diligence with which the exercises are performed, and thus the benefits derived as a result. It must be said, however, that so many people have enjoyed much better physical, mental and spiritual health as a result of Yoga that they have gone on to further exercises and more difficult and advanced postures. For that reason a short bibliography of helpful books on Yoga is given at the end of this book.

It will have been noticed that no actual "standing on one's head" exercises have been given here. Many people's view of Yoga is that of sitting on a bed of nails like a *fakir*, and then standing on one's head. There are head-standing exercises in Yoga (as the books recommended will show), but they are not given here for the simple reason that many people have not stood on their heads since they were made to do it as school-children and have a fear of dizziness, vertigo, fainting or falling. It is not a necessary Yoga exercise for the purposes of this book, and the Plough and the Shoulder-Stand come sufficiently near it to promote a flow of blood to the head. But let us take the exercises one by one and see how they can benefit us:

EXERCISE 1 (Sit-and-Breathe). This start at controlled breathing helps to impart a feeling of calmness and well-being. It helps to improve the circulation of the blood and increases resistance to colds and respiratory infections. It expands the chest and helps with voice production. Coupled with Exercises 2, 3, 4 and 5, these breathing exercises help to impart tranquillity and calmness and overcome nervousness and anxiety. Done immediately after some emotional upset, the benefits will be seen at once. Such breathing also helps to relieve headaches, and done last thing at night helps to overcome insomnia.

EXERCISES 6, 7, 8 and 21 (the Relaxation Exercises). In a fast-moving world, when everyone seems to be caught up in the "rat race," a world of noise and hustle and bustle, these relaxation exercises help us to attain freedom from too much tension. Some tension is desirable. No violin or guitar would produce music unless the strings were under tension! But too much tension results in the strings snapping! Relaxation helps us to be "in tune," at the "right pitch." In times when newspapers, radio and television feed other people's thoughts into our minds, we do not meditate and contemplate enough. During these relaxation moments we are in a position for such contemplation. It promotes patience, tolerance and endurance—qualities much-needed in our modern world.

EXERCISE 9 (the Leg-Pull). This exercise removes stiffness in the spine and tension in the neck and shoulders. At the same time the legs are greatly strengthened, which is of great advantage for preachers, shop assistants, schoolteachers, housewives, and so on.

EXERCISE 10 (the Leg-Flop). Again stiffness in the legs is eased away, especially in the thighs. The whole pelvic region is given a tonic when this exercise is completed. Like Exercise 9, it helps those who have to walk or stand for long periods.

EXERCISE 11 (the Backward Bend). This exercise again concentrates on the spine, giving it greater elasticity. At the same time it develops the chest and neck. The ankles and toes are also strengthened, as much of the weight of the body is upon them during this exercise.

EXERCISE 12 (On Your Toes). Toes, calves, thighs and the waist are helped by this posture. At the same time, balance and poise are practised. The whole of the waist and abdominal area improves through this posture.

EXERCISE 13 (Arm-and-Leg Triangle). As with Exercise 12, poise and balance are helped by this Arm-and-Leg Triangle. But it is much more than a graceful ballet dancer's stance. It stretches the spine, the knee joints and the ankle.

EXERCISE 14 (Chest Expander). Little-used shoulder muscles are strengthened with this exercise and the chest cage is expanded. The calf muscles are also toned up as the trunk is bent forward. This exercise is of great benefit to those whose daily occupation is a sedentary one.

EXERCISE 15 (the Upward-Press). Each vertebrae receives benefit from the stretching of the spine in this exercise. The chest is also strengthened. This is an excellent exercise for those who have suffered from a slipped disc.

EXERCISE 16 (the Leg-Lift). Again the slipped-disc or back sufferer will greatly benefit from this posture. New strength is gained in the lumbar region of the back. It also helps stimulate the liver, intestines, kidneys and other vital abdominal organs.

EXERCISE 17 (the Boat). Develops chest and thighs, strengthens the spine. Especially beneficial for slipped-disc sufferers.

EXERCISE 18 (the Neck-Twist). This exercise is a fine one for removing stiffness and tension of the neck. It is helpful to follow this exercise with a session of cross-legged sitting, at the same time turning the head slowly (with eyes closed) from left to right and right to left as far as it will go; then do the same up and down, beginning with the head on the chest; and finally perform circular movements with head, first clockwise, then anti-clockwise. Such movements provide wonderful relief from tightness and tension of the neck.

EXERCISE 19 (the Plough). The spine is again concentrated on in this exercise, the back being greatly strengthened, from neck to lumbar region.

EXERCISE 20 (the Shoulder-Stand). Helps to send blood headwards, revitalizing the brain. The internal organs are given a chance to "lean" in the opposite direction from normal. Shoulder, arm and back muscles are strengthened.

E

The only advice that need now be given is summed up in the two catch-phrases: "Three tries for a Welshman" and "If at first you don't succeed, try again!" Do not give up if you do not feel the above benefits after the first week or so of practice. Limbs will be stiff and muscles unused to working as they must do in these various exercises. But keep at it, daily, regularly, and the benefits will be felt by yourself and seen by others. After all, the Christian life, which we have seen is a life of discipline, is also a life of perseverance. Our forefathers in the faith used to talk about "the perseverance of the saints," in the sense that the truly converted man will be kept safe until he reaches heaven. There is another kind of Scriptural perseverance: "He that endureth to the end shall be saved" (Matthew 10: 22); and: "Love . . . beareth all things, believeth all things, hopeth all things, *endureth* all things" (1 Corinthians 13: 7). We are to "endure as good soldiers of Jesus Christ." So go on persevering in the practice of Yoga until the benefits are felt and seen; then you will not want to give it up, but rather others will take it up because of the conspicuous benefits you yourself have gained.

Chapter 7

VARIATIONS

W E HAVE SEEN that God is a God of order and design. He is also a God of infinite variety. The natural world around supplies abundant evidence to convince us. The constellations in the night sky; the pebbles on the sea-shore; the different species of fish, animals, birds, insects—all these and much else provide evidence of Divine variety.

Variety is often said to be "the spice of life." A life that knows no variety is dull and dreary. That is why "a change is as good as a rest." That is why we try to take an annual holiday. A change of scenery, people, atmosphere, and so on, all help us to come back and live in the daily round of common tasks.

Every athlete knows that rigorous training for an event can leave him "stale" unless he introduces some variety into his training schedule. He must run different distances at different speeds on different days. There must be periods of skipping or exercising. There must be a variation at several levels if he is to be in peak condition on the day of his event.

So every housewife who is intent on slimming knows that there must be variation in the slimming diet or she will soon begin to become averse to the diet and slip back into fattening foods.

In the same way the Yogi needs to vary his schedules occasionally so that he does not become stale. There are certain exercises that are more attractive than others, that appeal to us more. The danger is that we hasten through others to get to our favourite ones. The more difficult exercises sometimes become a drudgery instead of a delight. The solution is to introduce some variation into the schedules.

Before listing some books for further reading for those who have now become serious about Yoga and would like to go on and learn more difficult exercises, here are some variations of certain exercises already given. These variations make the simple, basic exercises slightly more strenuous and certainly more beneficial.

VARIATION 1 (for use with Kneel-and-Breathe, Exercise 3, and the Backward Bend, Exercise 11). Instead of the feet and toes pointing backwards in these two exercises the toes are curled under, the Yogi still sitting upon the heels.

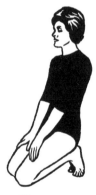

VARIATION 1

Varied with the more simple method already learned, this helps to strengthen feet and ankles. In the Backward Bend it makes the spine curve more, as it is farther back to reach the floor with the hands. For some time it will not be possible in the Backward Bend to place the palms of the hands flat on the floor, only the finger-tips.

VARIATION 2 (for use with the Leg-Pull, Exercise 9). By sitting as in Figure 1 below, the Leg-Pull can become the Alternate Leg-Pull. The one leg is tucked into the inside of the thigh of the other leg; both hands then reach out and clasp the ankle of the extended leg. Bending the elbows slightly outwards, the head is allowed to fall towards the knee of the extended leg. This exercise is done three times with each leg, holding the position for twenty seconds.

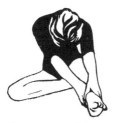

VARIATION 2. Fig. 1

Figure 2 below shows how the Leg-Pull can be varied a second time and the Leg-Pull can become the Complete Leg-Pull. The spine should be sufficiently supple now to enable the Yogi to grasp the soles or toes of the feet instead of merely the ankle. The same procedure of elbows

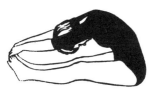

VARIATION 2. Fig. 2

outward and head bent to knees is followed, and the extreme position is held for twenty seconds.

VARIATION 3 (for use with the Leg-Lift, Exercise 16). Instead of both legs being lifted together they can now be raised one at a time. One leg lifted for five seconds, lowered; the next leg lifted for the same amount of time, lowered; then both legs lifted together. No diagram is needed to explain this simple variation of Exercise 16.

VARIATION 4 (for use with the Plough, Exercise 19). When the legs are lowered behind the head towards the floor as shown in Exercise 19, page 52, a variation is possible as illustrated below—that is, the legs are lowered wide apart.

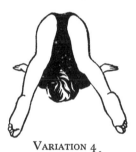

VARIATION 4.

VARIATION 5 (for use with the Shoulder-Stand, Exercise 20). Again, when the extreme position of the Shoulder-Stand is reached the legs can be allowed to go apart and be held in that position for the required number of seconds for Exercise 20.

These variations should now be "worked into" the schedules. The simple, basic exercise should be practised alternatively with the variation, not done one after the other in the same schedule. These variations will inspire the Yogi to go on to the more difficult exercises in the books recommended.

Chapter 8

THE EVERYDAY CHALLENGE

D R. EDWARD L. BORTZ has well said: "Physical fitness is the result of much more than mere physical activity. There is the need for a proper balance of a well-selected diet, adequate exercise, rest and recreation. The top essential is motivation: the individual must have a desire to keep himself physically fit. If the youth of a nation is flabby in mind as well as in body, what is the promise for the future of the older citizens?" There is here a daily challenge to young, middle-aged and older men and women. To achieve the well-being of body, mind and spirit described in the Introduction to this book, and to enjoy a full life, seven simple steps are all that is necessary.

First we must conquer our fear and reluctance. As Déchanet, the Benedictine monk who practises Yoga, declares: "It is not a question of turning a given form of Yoga into something Christian, but of bringing into the service of Christianity and of the Christian life the undoubted benefits arising from yogic discipline." With him we must see that Yoga postures are "neither more nor less peculiar than those in 'normal' physical culture, and familiar to many people." He uses strong language to help us overcome our fears: "There shall be no bastardy of compromise; but only a borrowing of methods, to be adapted immediately and introduced into an ascetic discipline authentically Christian in tenor and spirit." We are not concerned, as many Yogis are, with levitation, thought-reading, trance-states, or the suspension of certain vital powers, but rather with being Christians in the full sense of the word. Being "in Christ" we become *for* Christ without any half-measures or reservations. This is living victoriously.

The second step is to learn correct breathing. Again the Prior of Saint-André has a word for us: "It may seem odd or ridiculous or even absurd to stand on your head, and even more so to block your nostrils alternately in order to breathe. To the 'profane,' the exercises of Hatha Yoga are always amusing. None of them is spectacular in the sense of having something to show off when set beside the movements and turns of skill or strength in ordinary gymnastics. The Hatha Yoga exercises are carried out 'in single combat,' in silence and solitude; what, then, does it matter to the man doing the exercises if his attitudes look strange or his movements queer, when he derives benefit from them, and they result in a sense of physical and psychical regeneration?" The correct Yoga breathing is all-important. All the exercises or postures are of little use without the adoption of controlled breathing. Breathing correctly will promote a sense of peace and relaxation, and enable one to adopt the postures without fear of strain or falling.

Relaxation is the third step towards victory in everyday living. The Japanese version of the Twenty-third Psalm by Toki Miyashiro describes the victorious life of the Christian who has overcome strain and stress and is living in a relaxed state:

The Lord is my pace-setter, I shall not rush.
He makes me stop for quiet intervals; He provides me with images of stillness, which restore my serenity.
He leads me in ways of efficiency through calmness of mind, and His guidance is peace.

Even though I have a great many things to accomplish each day, I will not fret, for His presence is here.

His timelessness, His all-importance, will keep me in balance.

He prepares refreshment and renewal in the midst of my activity by anointing my mind with His oil of tranquillity, my cup of joyous energy overflows.

Surely harmony and effectiveness shall be the fruit of my hours, and I shall walk in the pace of the Lord, and dwell in His house for ever.

The postures constitute the fourth step. The adopting of these postures each day, some of them requiring balance, others bending of infrequently used parts of the body, results in a sense of yielding. The correct posture is only achieved after some effort has been exerted, but once achieved there is a stillness of body with the mind in tune. No haste, no unevenness, only simple and natural movements are necessary for these postures. There is no competitive spirit, as the postures are carried out in private, and "success" is an individual matter of accomplishment, not the striving after some tangible reward. This spirit of acceptance and achievement is reflected in our daily life, that life which is so complicated and competitive. No wonder it has been called a "rat race!"

The fifth step to victory is the faithful observance of the schedules. It is Yoga *every day* for Christians, not alternate days, or practise one day, miss the next. The time-tables must be adhered to and worked through correctly and consistently. Even if the schedules given in this book have to be modified, then the modified list of exercises *must* be practised each day. As Christians we are disciples of Christ. Disciple and discipline are two words that are very similar etymologically. A disciple is one who lives a disciplined life. Only a disciplined life is a victorious life.

Step six is to be on the look-out for the benefits. Yoga is beneficial to body, mind and spirit. For some, improvement may come first to the body, which will in turn affect the mind and spirit. For others, the mental outlook may improve, or one's spiritual life may improve in depth and growth. We would not copy some who make outlandish claims for Yoga—that it prolongs life well beyond the average span, or enables a mother to look younger than her daughter, or a father younger than his son! Every day that Yoga is practised by the Christian, however, he will discover that his body is benefiting from the exercises, his mind from the lack of tension, and his spirit through contemplation of Divine things.

The seventh step is variation. While the Christian lives a disciplined life, and in practising Yoga keeps to schedules and time-tables, he must never become the slave to routine. The nine-till-five routine that enslaves so many, sending them to another week's work with that "Monday-morning feeling," should never entrap the Christian who is practising Yoga. The variations introduced into the schedules set him free from routine, the "daily round and common task," making life pleasant and varied as it is meant to be.

Dr. Edward Bortz, past president of the American Medical Association, has said: "It begins to appear that exercise is the master conditioner for the healthy and the major therapy for the ill." The practice of Yoga as outlined in this book will provide that "conditioner" and that "therapy" that will help the under-exercised and the over-tensed.

Victorious living? Jesus Christ said that He came "that men may have life, and may have it *in all its fullness*" (John 10: 10, New English Bible). The Christian is one who has received the Divine Life by faith; he has become regenerate. To maintain that life in all its fullness, he must face life's daily demands, opportunities and problems truly "thinking success."

As Godfrey Robinson and Stephen Winward say in their book *The Art of Living*: "Get a *vision* of the great thing you want to accomplish. Get a *plan* of the way in which you hope to achieve it. Pray earnestly to God to give you the victory." It is hoped that this book will help many to catch the vision of victorious living; see God's plan for victorious living; and urge greater efforts in prayer to God for victorious living every day.

INDEX TO EXERCISES

In alphabetical order, not in order of practice.

BOOKS FOR FURTHER READING

Yoga

Alain: YOGA FOR PERFECT HEALTH (Thorsons Ltd., London).

Day: ABOUT YOGA (Brown Book Company, New York).

Déchanet: CHRISTIAN YOGA (Harper and Row, New York).

Hittleman: BE YOUNG WITH YOGA (Prentice-Hall, Inc., Englewood Cliffs, New Jersey.

Wood: PRACTICAL YOGA (Borden Publishing Company, Alhambra, California).

General

Beattie: THE HEART OF THINGS. Some Striking Analogies from Modern Medical Science. (Victory Press, London.)

Daily: RELEASE. Chapters on Relaxation, Concentration, and Meditation. (Arthur James, Evesham.)

Hutchinson: HIGHWAY TO HEALING, Part II for Private Devotion useful during Yoga exercises. (Arthur James, Evesham.)

ACKNOWLEDGMENTS

The author is indebted to the following publishers who have granted permission to use copyright material. However, should any such material have been used inadvertently without permission, then the author offers his apologies and promises to rectify the omission in any future edition of the book.

BOOK	PERMISSION FROM
Christian Yoga by Déchanet	Messrs. Burns & Oates Ltd. 25 Ashley Place London, S.W.1
	Messrs. Harper & Row Inc. 49 East 33rd Street New York U.S.A.
Creative Ageing by E. L. Bortz	The Macmillan Company 60 Fifth Avenue New York U.S.A.
The Art of Living by Godfrey Robinson and Stephen Winward	Messrs. Henry E. Walter Ltd. 26 Grafton Road Worthing Sussex

ACKNOWLEDGMENTS

The illustrations are by Geoffrey Venables of Worcester.